THE MIND DIET COOKBOOK COMPLETE GUIDE

A COMPREHENSIVE GUIDE TO EASY AND DELICIOUS HEALTHY EATING FOR NOURISHING MEALS THAT DELIGHT YOUR TASTE BUDS AND BOOST YOUR WELL-BEING

copyright@2024

Conklin Scott

TABLE OF CONTENT

INTRODUCTION

WHAT IS THE MIND DIET?

The MIND Diet, brief for Mediterranean Dash Diet Intervention for Neurodegenerative Delay, is a nutritional method designed to promote mind health and decrease the danger of neurodegenerative sicknesses like Alzheimer's. This food regimen combines elements of the Mediterranean and DASH (Dietary Approaches to Stop Hypertension) diets, focusing on foods that have been proven to assist cognitive characteristic and average brain fitness.

The MIND Diet emphasizes the consumption of mind boosting meals even as minimizing those related to cognitive decline. By incorporating loads of nutrient rich meals and proscribing much less healthy options, this food regimen pursuits to offer a practical, sustainable technique to keeping intellectual acuity as we age.

ORIGINS AND DEVELOPMENT

Developed through researchers at Rush University Medical Center, the MIND Diet emerged from substantial research linking dietary patterns to mind health. The food plan became formulated based totally on findings that certain foods and vitamins can positively effect mind feature, potentially reducing the danger of Alzheimer's sickness and different types of dementia.

KEY BENEFITS AND SCIENTIFIC EVIDENCE

Scientific studies helps the MIND Diet's potential to improve cognitive feature and sluggish cognitive decline. Key advantages include:

● Improved Brain Health: Studies show that adhering to the MIND Diet can also enhance memory and average cognitive function.

- Reduced Risk of Alzheimer's Disease: Research shows that the weight reduction plan may decrease the danger of developing Alzheimer's and other neurodegenerative situations.

- Support for Heart Health: Many meals emphasized with the aid of the MIND Diet are also beneficial for cardiovascular fitness, contributing to average properly being.

- This diet isn't always simply a fixed of dietary recommendations however a way of life approach aimed at fostering longtime period fitness and well being.

Why the MIND Diet?

In a international packed with complex diets and fleeting fitness developments, the MIND Diet stands out for its consciousness on each simplicity and effectiveness. Unlike more restrictive diets, it encourages a balanced approach to consuming that carries quite a few flavorful, nutritious ingredients. The MIND Diet is designed to be realistic, making it less difficult so that you can make lasting adjustments on your ingesting habits while enjoying a wide range of scrumptious meals.

KEY ADVANTAGES AND MEDICAL PROOF supporting the MIND weight reduction plan

Key Benefits and Scientific Evidence Supporting the MIND Diet

1. Improved Cognitive Function

One of the maximum enormous advantages of the MIND Diet is its potential to enhance cognitive feature. Studies have shown that people who adhere to the MIND Diet enjoy slower cognitive decline compared to people who observe less brain wholesome eating styles. Research posted in the journal Alzheimer's

Disease: Research shows that the eating regimen can also lower the hazard of growing Alzheimer's and other neurodegenerative conditions.

Support for Heart Health: Many ingredients emphasized through the MIND Diet also are beneficial for cardiovascular health, contributing to usual well being.

This food plan isn't always just a fixed of dietary hints but a lifestyle technique aimed toward fostering long term health and nicely being.

Why the MIND Diet?

In a global packed with complex diets and fleeting fitness trends, the MIND Diet stands out for its cognizance on each simplicity and effectiveness. Unlike greater restrictive diets, it encourages a balanced technique to consuming that includes a lot of flavorful, nutritious ingredients. The MIND Diet is designed to be sensible, making it easier on the way to make lasting adjustments for your eating habits even as taking part in a huge range of scrumptious meals.

In this cookbook, you'll find a wealth of recipes and pointers that will help you combine the MIND Diet into your every day lifestyles. From vibrant breakfasts to enjoyable dinners and healthy snacks, each recipe is crafted to guide your brain health even as delighting your taste buds. By following this guide, you're now not simply adopting a food regimen but embracing a way of life that nurtures your mind and average fitness.

Key blessings and medical proof helping the MIND eating regimen

Key Benefits and Scientific Evidence Supporting the MIND Diet

1. Improved Cognitive Function

One of the most great benefits of the MIND Diet is its capacity to decorate cognitive characteristic. Studies have proven that folks that adhere to the MIND Diet revel in slower cognitive decline as compared to those who comply with less brain healthful ingesting styles.

2. Reduced Risk of Alzheimer's Disease

The MIND Diet has been related to a decrease risk of Alzheimer's disorder and other kinds of dementia. A study conducted by the Rush University Medical Center, which became instrumental inside the development of the MIND Diet, discovered that people who adhered to the weight loss program had a 53% lower hazard of developing Alzheimer's. Even people who accompanied the weight loss program fairly noticed a large discount in hazard, about 35%.

3. Support for Heart Health

Many foods emphasized in the MIND Diet, such as leafy vegetables, nuts, and olive oil, are also useful for coronary heart fitness. The weight reduction plan's focus on reducing saturated fats and promoting unsaturated fats helps lower cholesterol levels and reduce the threat of cardiovascular disorder. The DASH (Dietary Approaches to Stop Hypertension) aspect of the MIND Diet specifically objectives heart health, presenting introduced cardiovascular benefits.

4. Anti Inflammatory and Antioxidant Effects

The MIND Diet includes foods wealthy in antioxidants and anti inflammatory compounds, such as berries, nuts, and inexperienced leafy veggies. These ingredients assist fight oxidative pressure and inflammation, which can be related to cognitive decline and neurodegenerative illnesses. Research shows that antioxidants play a critical role in defensive brain cells from damage and assisting universal mind health.

5. Enhanced Overall Well Being

Adopting the MIND Diet can result in stepped forward usual well being beyond just cognitive health. The weight loss plan's emphasis on entire, nutrientdense meals helps popular health, aids in weight control, and might lead to accelerated energy stages. For instance, entire grains and lean proteins provide sustained electricity, at the same time as healthy fats from nuts and olive oil contribute to a balanced mood and better standard health.

Scientific Evidence

● Rush University Medical Center Studies: Multiple studies from Rush University have established the MIND Diet's effectiveness in reducing the threat of Alzheimer's disease and slowing cognitive decline. The weight loss program's system changed into primarily based on tremendous research linking unique nutritional patterns to brain fitness.

- Journal of Alzheimer's Disease: A have a look at posted on this journal highlighted the MIND Diet's ability in decreasing cognitive decline, displaying that adherence to the eating regimen is related to a slower fee of cognitive aging.
- American Journal of Clinical Nutrition: Research featured in this journal helps the anti inflammatory and antioxidant blessings of the meals emphasized within the MIND Diet, reinforcing its function in helping brain fitness.

BENEFITS FOR COGNITIVE HEALTH AND GETTING OLD

Benefits for Cognitive Health and Aging

The MIND Diet gives several key benefits for cognitive health and ageing, making it a precious approach for promoting intellectual readability and reducing the chance of cognitive decline.

1. Slows Cognitive Decline

Adhering to the MIND Diet has been connected to a slower charge of cognitive decline. Studies, which include those from Rush University Medical Center, have found that people who observe the MIND Diet closely experience slower cognitive growing older compared to individuals who do no longer. This means that the food plan can assist keep intellectual sharpness and delay the onset of age related cognitive impairments.

2. Reduces the Risk of Alzheimer's Disease

The MIND Diet has been specifically related to a discounted threat of growing Alzheimer's ailment. Research suggests that folks that adhere to the MIND Diet have a substantially decrease chance of Alzheimer's compared to people who do now not. Even partial adherence to the diet has shown protecting effects, highlighting its ability as a preventative measure towards neurodegenerative diseases.

3. Enhances Memory and Learning

The nutrients emphasized inside the MIND Diet, along with antioxidants from berries and omega3 fatty acids from fish, assist brain capabilities like reminiscence and learning. Antioxidants help protect brain cells from oxidative strain, at the same time as omega3s are important for preserving healthy brain cellular membranes and selling cognitive characteristic.

4. Supports Overall Brain Health

The MIND Diet promotes the consumption of foods that assist typical brain fitness. For example, leafy greens, nuts, and entire grains provide critical vitamins, minerals, and wholesome fats that make a contribution to brain function. These vitamins play a position in retaining cognitive strategies and defensive in opposition to cognitive decline.

5. Improves Mood and Mental Well Being

Many of the meals protected inside the MIND Diet, consisting of nuts, seeds, and fish, were proven to have tremendous effects on temper and mental well being. Omega3 fatty acids, specifically, are recognized to influence temper regulation and might assist alleviate signs and symptoms of despair and anxiety.

CHAPTER 1: UNDERSTANDING THE MIND DIET

CORE PRINCIPLES

FOCUS ON BRAIN WHOLESOME FOODS

Focus on Brain Healthy Foods

The MIND Diet emphasizes eating a whole lot of mind wholesome ingredients which can be rich in nutrients regarded to assist cognitive function and typical brain health.

1. Leafy Greens

Examples: Spinach, kale, collard vegetables, swiss chard.

Benefits: Leafy vegetables are filled with vitamins and minerals, together with folate, nutrition K, and antioxidants. Vitamin K, particularly, is assumed to aid mind feature through promoting cognitive health and protective in opposition to cognitive decline. Antioxidants in leafy vegetables assist fight oxidative strain and infection, that are linked to neurodegenerative sicknesses.

2. Berries

Examples: Blueberries, strawberries, raspberries, blackberries.

Benefits: Berries are wealthy in antioxidants, in particular flavonoids, that have been proven to enhance reminiscence and put off mind getting older. They help lessen oxidative stress and infection inside the brain, that can contribute to better cognitive function and a decrease risk of cognitive decline.

3. Nuts

Examples: Walnuts, almonds, cashews, pistachios.

Benefits: Nuts are notable resources of healthful fats, which include omega3 fatty acids and polyunsaturated fats, that are essential for brain health. They also offer diet E, which has been related to a decrease risk of cognitive decline and stepped forward cognitive feature.

4. Whole Grains

 Examples: Brown rice, quinoa, complete wheat, oats.

 Benefits: Whole grains are rich in fiber, vitamins, and minerals that support normal health and brain feature. They help hold regular blood sugar levels, that is vital for cognitive health. The B nutrients discovered in whole grains are specifically beneficial for brain characteristic and energy production.

FOODS TO DEVOUR AND KEEP AWAY FROM

 Foods to Eat and Avoid on the MIND Diet The MIND Diet emphasizes the intake of brain healthy ingredients while limiting those that could negatively effect cognitive characteristic.

FOODS TO EAT

1. Leafy Greens

- Examples: Spinach, kale, collard greens, Swiss chard.

- Benefits: Rich in nutrients (particularly vitamin K), minerals, and antioxidants that aid brain fitness.

2. Berries

- Examples: Blueberries, strawberries, raspberries, blackberries.

- Benefits: Packed with antioxidants and flavonoid that enhance reminiscence and defend towards cognitive decline.

3. Nuts

- Examples: Walnuts, almonds, cashews, pistachios.

- Benefits: High in healthy fat, nutrition E, and antioxidants that aid mind feature and guard towards cognitive decline.

4. Whole Grains

- Examples: Brown rice, quinoa, complete wheat, oats.

- Benefits: Provide fiber, B nutrients, and steady power, assisting usual mind characteristic and health.

5. Fatty Fish

- Examples: Salmon, trout, sardines, mackerel.

- Benefits: Rich in omega three fatty acids which might be vital for retaining healthful brain cellular membranes and cognitive characteristic.

6. Olive Oil

- Benefits: Contains monounsaturated fats and antioxidants with anti inflammatory residences that guard mind cells and guide cognitive health.

7. Beans

- Examples: Lentils, chickpeas, black beans, kidney beans.

Benefits: High in fiber, protein, and vital nutrients like B vitamins and magnesium, which stabilize blood sugar and guide brain health.

8. Poultry

Examples: Chicken, turkey.

Benefits: Provides lean protein and nutrients inclusive of B nutrients and zinc that are essential for brain health.

9. Herbs and Spices

Examples: Turmeric, cinnamon, rosemary.

Benefits: Contain antioxidants and anti inflammatory compounds that help brain characteristic and health.

10. Red Wine (in Moderation)

Benefits: Contains restorative, an antioxidant that could offer neuroprotective outcomes, although it ought to be consumed sparsely.

Foods to Avoid

1. Red Meat

Examples: Beef, pork, lamb.

- Reasons: High in saturated fats and ldl cholesterol, which could negatively have an effect on mind health and boom the hazard of cognitive decline.

2. Butter and Margarine

- Reasons: High in saturated fat and trans fats, that can make a contribution to infection and cognitive decline.

3. Cheese

Examples: All types of cheese.

Reasons: High in saturated fats and cholesterol, that may negatively effect brain health.

4. Pastries and Sweets

Examples: Cakes, cookies, doughnuts.

Reasons: High in added sugars and dangerous fat, that could lead to inflammation and make a contribution to cognitive decline.

5. Fried Foods

Examples: French fries, fried bird, fried snacks.

Reasons: High in unhealthy fats and trans fats, that may negatively have an effect on mind fitness and increase the chance of cognitive problems.

6. Processed Foods

Examples: Packaged snacks, processed meats, equipped to consume food.

Reasons: Often excessive in bad fat, added sugars, and sodium, which can contribute to infection and cognitive decline.

7. High Sugar Beverages

Examples: Soda, sweetened juices, strength beverages.

Reasons: High in delivered sugars, that may lead to insulin resistance and irritation, negatively impacting mind health.

LIMITING RED MEAT, BUTTER, AND SUGARY FOODS

The MIND Diet recommends restricting sure meals to promote better cognitive fitness and decrease the threat of neurodegenerative illnesses.

1. Red Meat

Why Limit It:

- Saturated Fats: Red meat is excessive in saturated fats, that could contribute to irritation and cardiovascular troubles. Chronic irritation and poor cardiovascular health are connected to cognitive decline and an multiplied danger of Alzheimer's ailment.

- Cholesterol: High levels of cholesterol associated with beef intake can lead to atherosclerosis (hardening of the arteries), that may affect brain health and cognitive characteristic.

How to Limit It:

Reduce Frequency: Aim to restriction red meat consumption to 3 instances a month instead of numerous times a week.

Portion Control: When you do eat red meat, keep quantities small—ideally, no larger than three4 oz. In keeping with serving.

Choose Lean Cuts: Opt for lean cuts of red meat and trim seen fats earlier than cooking.

Alternatives:

Poultry: Chicken and turkey provide lean protein with decrease ranges of saturated fats.

Fish: Fatty fish like salmon and trout are rich in omega3 fatty acids useful for mind health.

Plant Based Proteins: Beans, lentils, and tofu are splendid alternatives that provide protein without the saturated fat of beef.

2. Butter

Why Limit It:

Saturated Fats: Butter is excessive in saturated fat, that could growth stages of LDL (bad) ldl cholesterol and make a contribution to irritation. High saturated fat consumption is connected to cognitive decline and improved chance of neurodegenerative illnesses.

Trans Fats: Some butter substitutes, like margarine, may also comprise trans fat, which can be even greater dangerous to mind fitness.

How to Limit It:

Use Sparingly: Minimize the use of butter in cooking and baking.

Opt for Alternatives: Use healthier fats inclusive of olive oil or avocado oil for cooking and baking.

Read Labels: If you operate margarine, choose options which are free from trans fats and high in unsaturated fats.

Alternatives:

Olive Oil: Rich in monounsaturated fat and antioxidants which are beneficial for brain fitness.

Avocado Oil: Another healthy fats choice with similar benefits to olive oil.

Nut Butters: Almond or peanut butter may be used sparsely as a substitute.

3. Sugary Foods

Why Limit It:

Added Sugars: Foods excessive in delivered sugars can lead to insulin resistance, infection, and expanded risk of growing type 2 diabetes—all of which can be related to a higher threat of cognitive decline and Alzheimer's sickness.

Blood Sugar Spikes: High sugar meals purpose speedy spikes and crashes in blood sugar degrees, that may have an effect on mood, strength stages, and cognitive feature.

How to Limit It:

- Avoid Sugary Beverages: Cut out or substantially reduce the consumption of sodas, sweetened teas, and electricity liquids.

- Limit Sweets: Reduce intake of goodies, desserts, cookies, and different sugary desserts.

- Check Labels: Be mindful of hidden sugars in packaged ingredients and choose products with lower sugar content material.

Alternatives:

- Fresh Fruits: Natural sweetness from end result gives crucial nutrients and fiber with out the brought sugars.

- Whole Grains: Choose complete grains like oatmeal or complete wheat products to meet cravings for some thing sweet and offer sustained power.

CHAPTER 2: SETTING UP FOR SUCCESS

KITCHEN PREPARATION

ESSENTIAL TOOLS AND GADGETS FOR THE MIND DIET KITCHEN

To effectively put together and experience meals on the MIND Diet, having the right tools and devices for your kitchen can make the process easier and more efficient.

1. High Quality Knives

Chef's Knife: Versatile for cutting, cutting, and dicing culmination, greens, and proteins.

Paring Knife: Ideal for peeling and specified cutting duties.

2. Cutting Boards

Multiple Boards: Use separate reducing boards for veggies and meats to prevent moveinfection.

Non Slip Mats: Ensure stability whilst cutting.

3. Measuring Cups and Spoons

Dry and Liquid Measuring Cups: For correct dimension of substances.

Measuring Spoons: Essential for specific dimension of spices and small portions.

4. Mixing Bowls

Variety of Sizes: Useful for blending substances, marinating, and getting ready salads.

Glass or Stainless Steel: Durable and nonreactive substances are preferred.

5. Food Processor

Multipurpose Processor: Great for reducing, cutting, shredding, and making sauces or dips.

6. Blender

High Powered Blender: Ideal for making smoothies, soups, and sauces. A blender with ice crushing capability is useful for smoothies and frozen treats.

7. Cookware

Non Stick Skillets: Useful for cooking with minimum oil, perfect for getting ready healthful dishes.

Saucepans and Stockpots: For cooking grains, beans, soups, and stews.

Baking Sheets and Pans: For roasting greens, baking fish, and other healthful dishes.

8. Slow Cooker or Instant Pot

Slow Cooker: Great for preparing hearty soups, stews, and beans with minimal attempt.

Instant Pot: Versatile for stress cooking, slow cooking, sauteing, and making yogurt.

9. Air Fryer

Air Fryer: Provides a more healthy way to experience crispy ingredients by means of the use of less oil as compared to standard frying.

10. Digital Food Scale

Food Scale: Useful for as it should be measuring ingredients, in particular when following recipes or component control.

MEAL PLANNING FOR THE MIND DIET

Effective meal making plans is essential for adhering to the MIND Diet and making sure you get the right vitamins to guide cognitive health. Here's a manual that will help you plan your meals, inclusive of pointers, strategies, and pattern meal ideas.

1. Understanding the MIND Diet Principles

Focus on Brain Healthy Foods: Emphasize leafy veggies, berries, nuts, entire grains, fatty fish, olive oil, beans, rooster, and herbs/spices.

Limit Less Healthy Foods: Minimize red meat, butter, cheese, pastries, fried foods, processed meals, and sugary liquids.

2. Planning Your Meals

Weekly Meal Planning:

1. Create a Meal Schedule:

- Breakfast: Plan nutrient rich options like smoothies with berries and spinach, or oatmeal with nuts and fruit.

- Lunch: Consider salads with leafy vegetables, beans, and lean protein, or whole grain bowls with veggies and fish.

- Dinner: Include plenty of dishes including grilled salmon with quinoa and vegetables, or a hearty bean stew with a side of leafy greens.

- Snacks: Prepare wholesome snacks like combined nuts, sparkling fruit, or yogurt with berries.

2. Make a Shopping List:

Produce: Leafy greens, berries, greens, culmination.

Proteins: Fatty fish, hen, beans.

Grains: Whole grains like brown rice, quinoa, oats.

Healthy Fats: Olive oil, nuts.

Others: Herbs, spices, and any pantry staples wanted.

3. Prepare a Weekly Menu:

Monday:

- Breakfast: Berry smoothie with spinach and flax seeds.

- Lunch: Quinoa salad with mixed greens, chickpeas, and a lemon vinaigrette.

- Dinner: Baked salmon with roasted Brussels sprouts and candy potatoes.

- Snack: A handful of walnuts and a small apple.

Tuesday:

- Breakfast: Overnight oats with blueberries and almonds.

- Lunch: Turkey and avocado wrap with a side of mixed vegetables.

- Dinner: Lentil soup with a facet of steamed kale.

- Snack: Carrot sticks with hummus.

Wednesday:

- Breakfast: Greek yogurt with strawberries and a sprinkle of chia seeds.

- Lunch: Bean and vegetable stirfry over brown rice.

- Dinner: Grilled chicken with a quinoa and vegetable salad.

- Snack: A small handful of combined nuts.

Thursday:

- Breakfast: Whole grain toast with avocado and a facet of sparkling fruit.

- Lunch: Spinach and berry salad with grilled hen.
- Dinner: Turkey chili with a aspect of sautéed greens.
- Snack: Sliced bell peppers with a yogurt dip.

Friday:

- Breakfast: Smoothie bowl with blended berries, spinach, and a sprinkle of nuts.
- Lunch: Mediterranean chickpea salad with olive oil dressing.
- Dinner: Baked cod with roasted greens and a aspect of quinoa.
- Snack: An orange and a handful of almonds.

CHAPTER 3: BREAKFASTS

QUICK AND NUTRITIOUS OPTIONS

SMOOTHIES AND BOWLS WITH BERRIES AND NUTS

Incorporating berries and nuts into smoothies and bowls is an brilliant way to create nutrient dense, mind wholesome meals. Both components are wealthy in antioxidants, healthful fats, and critical nutrients that help cognitive characteristic.

Smoothies

1. Berry Spinach Smoothie

Ingredients:

1 cup clean spinach

half cup blueberries

half of cup strawberries (fresh or frozen)

1 banana

1 cup unsweetened almond milk (or any favored milk)

1 tablespoon chia seeds

1 tablespoon almond butter

Instructions:

1. Combine all components in a blender.

2. Blend until easy.

3. Pour into a pitcher and revel in straight away.

2. Berry Banana Smoothie

Ingredients:

1/2 cup raspberries

half cup blackberries

1 banana

1 cup Greek yogurt (simple or vanilla)

1 tablespoon flax seeds

half cup water or almond milk (alter for desired consistency)

Instructions:

1. Add all ingredients to a blender.

2. Blend until smooth and creamy.

3. Serve chilled.

3. Nutty Berry Smoothie

 Ingredients:

   1 cup combined berries (blueberries, strawberries, raspberries)

   1 tablespoon peanut butter or almond butter

   half cup low fat milk or plant based totally milk

   1/2 cup undeniable Greek yogurt

   1 tablespoon honey or maple syrup (elective)

   1/four cup chopped nuts (e.G., almonds, walnuts)

OVERNIGHT OATS WITH SEEDS AND FRUITS

Overnight oats are a convenient and nutritious breakfast alternative that may be easily customized to suit your flavor options and dietary wishes.

BASIC OVERNIGHT OATS RECIPE

Ingredients:

half cup rolled oats

1/2 cup milk (dairy or plant based totally, along with almond or soy milk)

half of cup Greek yogurt (plain or vanilla)

1 tablespoon chia seeds

1 tablespoon flax seeds

1 tablespoon honey or maple syrup (optional)

1/2 teaspoon vanilla extract (optional)

Instructions:

1. In a jar or hermetic container, integrate the rolled oats, milk, Greek yogurt, chia seeds, and flax seeds.

2. Stir in honey or maple syrup and vanilla extract if preferred.

Three. Mix properly until all ingredients are combined.

Four. Cover and refrigerate in a single day (or for at the least 4 hours).

5. In the morning, stir the oats and top together with your favourite culmination and nuts.

Flavor Variations and AddIns

1. Berry Bliss Overnight Oats

Toppings: Fresh blueberries, sliced strawberries, and raspberries.

Additional Seeds: 1 tablespoon of hemp seeds.

Instructions: After refrigerating in a single day, pinnacle with fresh berries and a sprinkle of hemp seeds.

2. Apple Cinnamon Overnight Oats

Toppings: Chopped apple, a sprinkle of cinnamon, and a handful of walnuts.

Instructions: Add 1/four teaspoon of floor cinnamon to the oats aggregate before refrigerating. In the morning, top with chopped apples and walnuts.

3. Tropical Overnight Oats

Toppings: Diced mango, pineapple, and a sprinkle of shredded coconut.

Additional Seeds: 1 tablespoon of chia seeds.

Instructions: Mix in some diced mango and pineapple with the oats aggregate earlier than refrigerating. Top with shredded coconut in the morning.

4. Nutty Banana Overnight Oats

Toppings: Sliced banana, chopped almonds, and a drizzle of almond butter.

Instructions: Add 1 tablespoon of almond butter to the oats combination earlier than refrigerating. In the morning, pinnacle with sliced banana and chopped almonds.

5. Peach Almond Overnight Oats

Toppings: Diced peaches and a sprinkle of slivered almonds.

Instructions: Mix 1/four cup of diced peaches into the oats combination before refrigerating. Top with slivered almonds inside the morning.

WHOLE GRAIN TOASTS WITH AVOCADO

Whole grain toasts with avocado are a simple but versatile dish that may be enjoyed for breakfast, lunch, or as a snack. They are nutritious, satisfying, and align nicely with the MIND Diet ideas. Here's how to put together primary avocado toast and a few scrumptious versions:

BASIC AVOCADO TOAST

Ingredients:

12 slices of entire grain bread

1 ripe avocado

Salt and pepper to flavor

Optional: Red pepper flakes, lemon juice, or olive oil

Instructions:

1. Toast the Bread: Toast the whole grain bread on your favored level of crispiness.

2. Prepare the Avocado: Cut the avocado in half, dispose of the pit, and scoop the flesh right into a bowl.

Three. Mash the Avocado: Mash the avocado with a fork till clean, leaving some chunks if desired.

Four. Season: Season the mashed avocado with salt and pepper. For greater taste, add a pinch of red pepper flakes, a squeeze of lemon juice, or a drizzle of olive oil.

Five. Assemble: Spread the mashed avocado flippantly over the toasted bread.

6. Serve: Enjoy at once.

FLAVOR VARIATIONS AND TOPPINGS

1. Tomato and Basil Avocado Toast

Toppings: Sliced cherry tomatoes, sparkling basil leaves, a drizzle of balsamic glaze.

Instructions: Top the avocado toast with sliced cherry tomatoes and fresh basil leaves. Drizzle with balsamic glaze.

2. Egg and Spinach Avocado Toast

Toppings: A poached or scrambled egg, sparkling spinach leaves.

Instructions: Top the avocado toast with a poached or scrambled egg and a handful of fresh spinach.

3. Smoked Salmon Avocado Toast

Toppings: Sliced smoked salmon, capers, a sprinkle of dill.

Instructions: Top the avocado toast with sliced smoked salmon, capers, and a sprinkle of fresh dill.

4. Red Pepper and Feta Avocado Toast

Toppings: Sliced roasted red peppers, crumbled feta cheese.

Instructions: Top the avocado toast with sliced roasted red peppers and crumbled feta cheese.

5. Apple and Almond Avocado Toast

Toppings: Thinly sliced apple, chopped almonds, a drizzle of honey.

Instructions: Top the avocado toast with thinly sliced apple and chopped almonds. Drizzle with honey.

CHAPTER 4: LUNCHES

SALADS AND BOWLS

LEAFY GREENS WITH LEAN PROTEINS

Combining leafy greens with lean proteins creates nutrient rich meals that support ordinary health and cognitive feature, specially in step with the MIND Diet.

1. Spinach and Chicken Salad

Ingredients:

2 cups fresh spinach

1 cup cooked, diced fowl breast

1/2 cup cherry tomatoes, halved

1/four cup sliced cucumbers

1/4 cup red onion, thinly sliced

2 tablespoons balsamic vinaigrette or lemon juice

Salt and pepper to taste

Instructions:

1. Prepare the Salad: In a massive bowl, combine the spinach, cooked chicken, cherry tomatoes, cucumbers, and pink onion.

2. Dress: Drizzle with balsamic French dressing or lemon juice. Toss to coat frivolously.

3. Season: Add salt and pepper to taste.

4. Serve: Enjoy right away or sit back till ready to serve.

2. Kale and Turkey Stir Fry

Ingredients:

2 cups chopped kale

1 cup cooked floor turkey

1 bell pepper, sliced

1 small onion, chopped

2 cloves garlic, minced

1 tablespoon olive oil

1 tablespoon soy sauce or tamari

1 teaspoon grated ginger

Salt and pepper to flavor

SOUPS AND STEWS

Soups and stews are comforting, nutritious, and flexible food that may be tailored to the MIND Diet standards. They're ideal for incorporating quite a few vegetables, lean proteins, and entire grains.

1. Lentil and Vegetable Soup

Ingredients:

1 cup dried lentils (rinsed and tired)

2 tablespoons olive oil

1 onion, chopped

2 cloves garlic, minced

2 carrots, diced

2 celery stalks, diced

1 pink bell pepper, diced

1 can (14.Five ounces) diced tomatoes

4 cups vegetable broth

1 teaspoon dried thyme

1 teaspoon ground cumin

Salt and pepper to taste

2 cups chopped kale or spinach

Instructions:

1. Heat Oil: In a huge pot, heat olive oil over medium warmness. Add onion and garlic, and prepare dinner till softened.

2. Add Vegetables: Stir in carrots, celery, and bell pepper. Cook for 57 minutes.

3. Add Lentils and Broth: Add lentils, diced tomatoes, and vegetable broth. Stir in thyme and cumin. Bring to a boil.

Four. Simmer: Reduce heat and simmer for 30forty mins, or till lentils are soft.

Five. Add Greens: Stir in kale or spinach and cook dinner until wilted.

6. Season: Add salt and pepper to taste.

7. Serve: Enjoy hot.

 2. Chicken and Spinach Stew

Ingredients:

 1 lb chicken breast or thighs, cut into bite sized portions

 2 tablespoons olive oil

 1 onion, chopped

2 cloves garlic, minced

2 carrots, sliced

1 zucchini, diced

1 cup sparkling spinach

4 cups fowl broth

1 teaspoon dried oregano

1 teaspoon dried basil

Salt and pepper to flavor

Instructions:

1. Cook Chicken: In a big pot, warmness olive oil over medium warmth. Add fowl pieces and cook dinner till browned.

2. Add Aromatics: Add onion and garlic, and prepare dinner till softened.

3. Add Vegetables and Broth: Stir in carrots, zucchini, and hen broth. Add oregano and basil. Bring to a boil.

4. Simmer: Reduce warmness and simmer for 20halfhour, or till bird is cooked thru and greens are soft.

5. Add Spinach: Stir in spinach and prepare dinner till wilted.

6. Season: Add salt and pepper to flavor.

7. Serve: Enjoy warm.

3. Sweet Potato and Black Bean Chili

Ingredients:

 1 tablespoon olive oil

 1 onion, chopped

 2 cloves garlic, minced

 1 purple bell pepper, diced

 1 green bell pepper, diced

 2 medium sweet potatoes

LENTIL AND VEGETABLE SOUPS

Lentil and vegetable soups are a brilliant option for a hearty, nutritious meal. They're rich in fiber, protein, and important vitamins whilst being flexible and smooth to put together.

 1. Classic Lentil and Vegetable Soup

Ingredients:

1 cup dried inexperienced or brown lentils, rinsed

2 tablespoons olive oil

1 onion, chopped

2 cloves garlic, minced

2 carrots, diced

2 celery stalks, diced

1 crimson bell pepper, diced

1 can (14.Five oz) diced tomatoes

4 cups vegetable broth

1 teaspoon dried thyme

1 teaspoon floor cumin

1 bay leaf

Salt and pepper to flavor

2 cups chopped kale or spinach (elective)

Instructions:

1. Heat Oil: In a large pot, warmness olive oil over medium warmth. Add onion and garlic, and cook dinner till softened.

2. Add Vegetables: Stir in carrots, celery, and bell pepper. Cook for approximately 5 minutes.

3. Add Lentils and Broth: Add lentils, diced tomatoes, and vegetable broth. Stir in thyme, cumin, and bay leaf.

4. Simmer: Bring to a boil, then lessen heat and simmer for 3040 mins, or till lentils are smooth.

5. Add Greens (Optional): Stir in kale or spinach and prepare dinner till wilted.

6. Season: Add salt and pepper to flavor. Remove bay leaf earlier than serving.

7. Serve: Enjoy warm.

TOMATO AND FISH STEWS

Tomato and fish stews are flavorful and nutrient packed dishes which might be each pleasant and wholesome. They combine the wealthy taste of tomatoes with the lightness of fish, developing a balanced meal.

1. Mediterranean Tomato and Fish Stew

Ingredients:

1 lb white fish fillets (such as cod, haddock, or tilapia), cut into chunks

2 tablespoons olive oil

1 onion, chopped

2 cloves garlic, minced

1 crimson bell pepper, diced

1 can (14.Five oz) diced tomatoes

1 cup fish or vegetable broth

1 teaspoon dried oregano

1 teaspoon dried basil

half of teaspoon smoked paprika

Salt and pepper to flavor

1/four cup chopped Kalamata olives (optional)

1 tablespoon capers (optional)

Fresh parsley for garnish

Instructions:

1. Heat Oil: In a big pot, warmth olive oil over medium warmth. Add onion and garlic, and cook dinner till softened.

2. Add Vegetables: Stir in bell pepper and prepare dinner for approximately five minutes.

3. Add Tomatoes and Broth: Add diced tomatoes and broth. Stir in oregano, basil, and smoked paprika.

4. Simmer: Bring to a boil, then lessen warmness and simmer for 10 mins.

5. Add Fish: Gently add fish chunks to the pot. Simmer for 1015 minutes, or until fish is cooked through and flakes without difficulty.

6. Add Olives and Capers (Optional): Stir in olives and capers if the use of.

7. Season: Add salt and pepper to taste.

8. Serve: Garnish with fresh parsley and serve warm.

CHAPTER 5: DINNERS

MAIN COURSES

RECIPES FEATURING FISH AND POULTRY

Combining fish and fowl in meals can offer a fantastic balance of lean protein, healthful fat, and vital vitamins.

1. Chicken and Salmon Bake

Ingredients:

2 fowl breasts

2 salmon fillets

2 tablespoons olive oil

1 lemon, sliced

1 teaspoon dried thyme

1 teaspoon dried rosemary

1 garlic clove, minced

Salt and pepper to taste

1 cup cherry tomatoes, halved

1 cup child potatoes, halved

Instructions:

1. Preheat Oven: Preheat your oven to four hundred°F (2 hundred°C).

2. Prepare Chicken: Rub bird breasts with olive oil, thyme, rosemary, garlic, salt, and pepper.

3. Prepare Salmon: Rub salmon fillets with olive oil, salt, and pepper.

4. Arrange: Place fowl breasts and salmon fillets on a baking sheet. Surround with cherry tomatoes and infant potatoes.

5. Add Lemon: Top hen and salmon with lemon slices.

6. Bake: Bake for 2530 minutes, or until chicken reaches an internal temperature of 165°F (seventy four°C) and salmon is cooked thru.

7. Serve: Serve hot with a facet of steamed vegetables or a clean salad.

 2. Chicken and Fish Tacos

Ingredients:

1 lb chicken breast, diced

half of lb white fish fillets (inclusive of cod), diced

2 tablespoons olive oil

1 teaspoon ground cumin

1 teaspoon paprika

half teaspoon chili powder

Salt and pepper to taste

eight small corn tortillas

1 cup shredded cabbage

half of cup diced tomatoes

1/four cup chopped cilantro

Lime wedges for serving

Instructions:

1. Season and Cook Chicken: In a skillet, heat olive oil over medium warmness. Add diced bird, cumin, paprika, chili powder, salt, and pepper. Cook till chook is no longer purple and cooked through.

2. Cook Fish: In the identical skillet, upload a chunk more olive oil if wished and prepare dinner diced fish until opaque and flaky.

3. Assemble Tacos: Warm tortillas and fill with a combination of hen and fish.

Four. Top: Top with shredded cabbage, diced tomatoes, and chopped cilantro.

5. Serve: Serve with lime wedges for squeezing over the pinnacle.

3. Fish and Chicken Skewers

Ingredients:

1 lb chicken breast, reduce into chunks

1/2 lb firm white fish fillets, cut into chunks

1 red bell pepper, cut into chunks

1 green bell pepper, cut into chunks

1 onion, reduce into chunks

2 tablespoons olive oil

1 tablespoon lemon juice

VEGETABLE AND GRAIN BASED DISHES

Vegetable and grain based dishes are nutritious, versatile, and can be both hearty and fulfilling. They provide a great manner to experience lots of vegetables and entire grains.

1. Quinoa and Roasted Vegetable Salad

Ingredients:

1 cup quinoa, rinsed

2 cups water or vegetable broth

1 cup cherry tomatoes, halved

1 zucchini, diced

1 pink bell pepper, diced

1 cup diced butternut squash

2 tablespoons olive oil

1 teaspoon dried oregano

Salt and pepper to taste

1/four cup crumbled feta cheese (optional)

2 tablespoons balsamic French dressing

Fresh basil for garnish

Instructions:

1. Cook Quinoa: In a medium saucepan, carry water or vegetable broth to a boil. Add quinoa, lessen warmth, and simmer for 15 mins, or till quinoa is cooked and water is absorbed. Fluff with a fork and allow cool.

2. Roast Vegetables: Preheat oven to 425°F (220°C). Toss cherry tomatoes, zucchini, bell pepper, and butternut squash with olive oil, oregano, salt, and pepper. Spread on a baking sheet and roast for 2025 mins, or till gentle and barely caramelized.

Three. Combine: In a big bowl, mix cooked quinoa with roasted vegetables. Add feta cheese if using.

4. Dress: Drizzle with balsamic French dressing and toss to mix.

5. Serve: Garnish with fresh basil and serve warm or at room temperature.

 2. Chickpea and Spinach Stew

Ingredients:

1 tablespoon olive oil

1 onion, chopped

2 cloves garlic, minced

1 can (15 oz.) chickpeas, tired and rinsed

1 can (14.Five oz.) diced tomatoes

1 cup vegetable broth

1 teaspoon floor cumin

1 teaspoon smoked paprika

half teaspoon turmeric

half of teaspoon ground coriander

2 cups clean spinach

Salt and pepper to taste

Fresh cilantro for garnish

Instructions:

1. Cook Aromatics: In a big pot, heat olive oil over medium heat. Add onion and garlic and cook dinner till softened.

2. Add Spices: Stir in cumin, paprika, turmeric, and coriander, and cook dinner for 1 minute.

3. Add Chickpeas and Tomatoes: Add chickpeas, diced tomatoes, and vegetable broth. Bring to a boil.

Four. Simmer: Reduce warmness and simmer for 15 minutes to permit flavors to meld.

5. Add Spinach: Stir in spinach and cook till wilted.

6. Season: Add salt and pepper to taste.

7. Serve: Garnish with fresh cilantro and serve hot.

3. Barley and Vegetable Stir Fry

Ingredients:

1 cup pearl barley

2 cups water or vegetable broth

2 tablespoons olive oil

1 onion, chopped

2 cloves garlic, minced

1 cup broccoli florets

1 purple bell pepper, sliced

1 cup snap peas

2 tablespoons soy sauce or tamari

1 tablespoon rice vinegar

1 teaspoon sesame oil

1/four cup chopped inexperienced onions

Sesame seeds for garnish (optionally available)

DELICIOUS SIDE DISHES

Side dishes can supplement major guides or function a standalone mild meal.

1. Roasted Brussels Sprouts with Balsamic Glaze

Ingredients:

1 lb Brussels sprouts, trimmed and halved

2 tablespoons olive oil

1 tablespoon balsamic vinegar

1 tablespoon honey or maple syrup

Salt and pepper to taste

1/four cup shaved Parmesan cheese (elective)

Instructions:

1. Preheat Oven: Preheat your oven to 425°F (220°C).

2. Prepare Brussels Sprouts: Toss Brussels sprouts with olive oil, salt, and pepper.

3. Roast: Spread on a baking sheet and roast for 2025 mins, or till crispy and caramelized.

4. Prepare Glaze: In a small saucepan, combine balsamic vinegar and honey. Simmer over medium warmness until decreased and thickened.

Five. Finish: Drizzle roasted Brussels sprouts with balsamic glaze and sprinkle with Parmesan cheese if the use of.

ROASTED VEGETABLES

Roasting vegetables brings out their natural sweetness and complements their flavors.

1. Classic Roasted Vegetables

Ingredients:

1 large purple bell pepper, chopped

1 large yellow bell pepper, chopped

1 big zucchini, sliced

1 huge carrot, peeled and sliced

1 pink onion, chopped

2 tablespoons olive oil

1 teaspoon dried thyme

1 teaspoon dried rosemary

Salt and pepper to flavor

Instructions:

1. Preheat Oven: Preheat your oven to 425°F (220°C).

2. Prepare Vegetables: In a large bowl, toss bell peppers, zucchini, carrot, and pink onion with olive oil, thyme, rosemary, salt, and pepper.

3. Roast: Spread greens on a baking sheet in a unmarried layer. Roast for 25halfhour, stirring halfway via, till vegetables are smooth and lightly caramelized.

4. Serve: Serve heat as a side dish or over a bed of quinoa or rice.

 2. Mediterranean Roasted Vegetables

Ingredients:

1 cup cherry tomatoes

1 cup infant potatoes, halved

1 cup eggplant, diced

1 cup bell peppers (mixed shades), chopped

2 tablespoons olive oil

1 tablespoon dried oregano

1 teaspoon garlic powder

Salt and pepper to taste

1/four cup crumbled feta cheese (non compulsory)

Fresh basil for garnish

Instructions:

1. Preheat Oven: Preheat your oven to 425°F (220°C).

2. Prepare Vegetables: In a huge bowl, toss cherry tomatoes, baby potatoes, eggplant, and bell peppers with olive oil, oregano, garlic powder, salt, and pepper.

3. Roast: Spread veggies on a baking sheet in a unmarried layer. Roast for 2530 minutes, stirring midway via.

4. Finish: Sprinkle with crumbled feta cheese if desired and garnish with sparkling basil.

5. Serve: Serve heat as a aspect dish or a topping for salads.

3. Honey Glazed Roasted Carrots

Ingredients:

1 lb carrots, peeled and reduce into sticks

2 tablespoons olive oil

2 tablespoons honey

1 teaspoon dried thyme

Salt and pepper to flavor

Fresh parsley for garnish (elective)

Instructions:

1. Preheat Oven: Preheat your oven to four hundred°F (two hundred°C).

2. Prepare Carrots: In a massive bowl, toss carrots with olive oil, honey, thyme, salt, and pepper.